How to Adjust Yourself and Avoid Seeing a Chiropractor

By

Dr. Staten "C" Medsker, Jr.

(aka Rockndoc)

DrStatenMedsker.com

ROCKNDOC

Live Well & Rock On!

How to Adjust Yourself and Avoid Seeing a Chiropractor

Copyright @ 2020 by Dr. Staten "C" Medsker, Jr.

Published in the United States by BCG Publishing, 2020.

www.BCGPublishing.com

Disclaimer

The following viewpoints in this book are those of Dr. Staten "C" Medsker, Jr. These views are based on his personal experience over the past fifty-six years on the planet Earth, especially while living in the United States of America.

The intention of this book is to share his story about creating a new exercise program (S.E.T. Program) for musicians, professional athletes and the general public and what has worked for them through this journey.

All attempts have been made to verify the information provided by this publication. Neither the author nor the publisher assumes any responsibility for errors, omissions, or contrary interpretations of the subject matter herein.

This book is for entertainment purposes only. The views expressed are those of the author alone and should not be taken as expert instruction or commands. The reader is responsible for his or her future action. This book makes no guarantees of future success. However, by following the steps that are listed in this book the odds of obtaining correction of skeletal imbalances and achieving optimum health have a much higher probability.

Neither the author nor the publisher assumes any responsibility or liability on the behalf of the purchaser or reader of these materials.

The views expressed are based on his personal experiences within the corporate world, education, and everyday life.

This book is dedicated to my dad, Staten Medsker, Sr. Whom with his 3 failed low back surgeries and suffering daily agonizing pain would not have motivated me to continue to search for alternative therapies throughout my education and professional life. To my mother, Bonnie Jean Butz who is an icon and example of pure love and service for all the individuals in her community. To my wife, Courtney Louise Medsker-Drake who proves to me everyday that there are positive outcomes to every challenge put upon us by being patient, understanding and empathetic and she is one of the greatest mothers I've ever witnessed in parenting our 3-year-old, Presley.

I am also dedicating this book to every musician and patient that I have had the privilege working with in helping me create this S.E.T. Program. Your dedication for physical change, allowing me to ride on the coat tails of your fame and your drive for success and trying new things have all gone above and beyond the standard call of duty and devotion and I am proud and honored to be able to help you in your journey.

Table of Contents

FOREWORD BY JO FASEN
MPT, OCS, CSCS, CERT. MDT

I met Dr. Medsker in early 2017. I walked into his office, having never met him, to see if he wanted to collaborate on a project I was working on; from a healthcare and expert in his field colleague perspective. Out of that chance visit, I benefited and learned much more than I anticipated. I am a Physical Therapist (PT) involved in several healthcare leadership roles and initiatives and have had the pleasure working with many chiropractors over my 26-year career. I have been both a colleague and a patient of chiropractors. I admit being quite particular with which medical professionals I associate with and feel qualified in knowing a great practitioner when I see one. Dr. Medsker is truly unique and skilled in his craft. I was immediately impressed with his welcoming, giving, kind, compassionate and sharing spirit. It was clear he had a following. His office was filled with sunlight coming through the windows that paled in comparison to the light he gave off with his positive energy and expression of authentic passion for what he does to help his patients move better and feel better. The walls were covered with photos of the many he helps and who travel far to see him. It was not hard to see Dr. Medsker was a <u>gifted healer</u> and I wanted to hear more.

It's fun to hear he is the "Doc" to the musical stars and many other notables of our time, but I soon found out Dr. Medsker is not a "one trick pony". You name it, he is sought after for his <u>gifted healing</u> and gets results with all populations.

Our goal is to empower patients, giving them the tools, to learn and perform their individualized programs for long term healing results. As a PT, I know how important it is to not only teach and perform truths about treatment protocols but also how difficult it is to get patient compliance to follow the home programs that we design for our patients. My mantra of "you can't take me home with you" is not always enough to motivate one to take committed action with their program. Dr. Medsker's S.E.T Program is very easy to follow, commit to, and gets results. Let's face it, if it's not simple and convenient people are not likely to do it or do it for life for general maintenance; which is many times necessary. This program meets that criteria and can be done in the convenience of one's home, home on the road, or gym. I quickly appreciated Dr. Medsker and I shared a very aligned language.

I feel the need to practice what I preach so I was eager to check out this S.E.T. Program. Having benefited from PT and Chiropractic care, and knowing I have many alignment issues from "life" and past sports injuries; trying this was a no-brainer. I, like many of you, had way too much on my plate and could really test if it was easy and convenient. Bring it on. I applied most of the S.E.T. Program (combined with some of my own PT self-care stuff that was complimentary) and felt the results. It wasn't until I suffered a recent bike accident that I continued to experience even greater results.

I was biking to work and by an unexpected freak of nature a large branch got caught in my back tire spoke throwing me violently onto the cement fracturing my right pelvis in multiple places. It didn't take much to figure I would likely have more alignment issues now. I was confined to a wheelchair many weeks, followed by the progression to walkers, crutches, and canes as my healing progressed. Due to the extended distance and inability to travel, I was forced to do most of my treatment by myself at home. Utilizing my own expertise and combining Dr. Medsker's S.E.T Program, I have healed much quicker and saved hundreds of dollars on would be office visits. As soon as I could drive myself and my fractures stabilized more, I headed to Dr. Medsker to assess the damage to my alignment and peripheral tissues impacted by the crash.

Dr. Medsker was instrumental in my healing as we were able to do regular leg length measurements to track the ongoing healing of my fractured pelvis and its surrounding soft tissues. Early on and throughout my healing I stretched throughout the day, every day, and used the pelvic blocks 3x a day or more. We saw a large reduction of my leg length from 18mm to 4mm in a short period of time (approximately 3 months). I also perform the self-adjusting stretches and positions feeling the vertebra respond and my soft tissue lengthen, occasionally hearing that audible "pop" validating I'm "moving" in the right direction. Now my job is to continue and maintain that, of course, but again, it's easy and convenient, so I'm in. And it works.

I would recommend this book to anyone experiencing back and neck pain but more so to anyone experiencing no pain. This information is great to prevent pain as well. It is a known researched fact that underlying skeletal compensations and imbalances exist in most everyone, and they are not symptomatic. In hopes of keeping it that way, this book has the potential in the prevention of spine and soft tissue related pain. I think of it as a movement "vitamin". We surely benefit from technology and smart phone advancements, but with them we are seeing the development of faultier postural and soft tissue problematic imbalances that can easily become painful. This book goes a long way in addressing what one can do for the increasing physical stressors we are exposing ourselves to.

In summary, I am confident you will find some personal benefit in reading this book and learning about what you can do to care for yourself. It applies alone or as a compliment to your care with a Chiropractor, PT, or related practitioner. Read it, apply it, even a few of the suggestions, and even if you have not sustained a brutal bike accident. You too, can enjoy the benefits of moving and feeling better through Dr. Medsker's healing wisdom and advice.

Jo Fasen, MPT, OCS, CSCS, Cert. MDT

Masters in Physical Therapy; Board Certified Orthopedic Clinical Specialist; Certified Strength and Conditioning Specialist and Certified in Mechanical Diagnosis and Therapy (Multi-specialty clinician, Clinic Director, Educator, Mentor, Advocate and Community Volunteer)

INTRODUCTION

In my 30 years of practice, all I tried to do was to teach my patients how to be more proactive in their care. The old cliché "if you feed a man a fish, you feed him for a day. If you teach a man to fish, then you feed him for a lifetime" has been my motto from the start. I found myself forced into creating a program for all my musician patients who were on tour. I got tired of putting so much effort into correcting their problems while they were here at home, only to lose all the work we did while they went out on the road. This is the program I was inspired to create to empower my patients to self-healing and educating them to get the most work done in the shortest amount of time while on their tour bus or different hotel rooms. The life of a rockstar is very fast paced and physically demanding on the human frame.

In this book you will learn not only how to stretch your body effectively to get the best outcome of flexibility but also how to adjust your own body (and others) the proper way to unlock any joints that have been stuck over the years. You will also find proper traction fulcrums and positioning so you obtain lasting structural changes that will give you more stability in your frame than you've ever had before in your life.

I have tried and proven this "S.E.T. Program" under such stressors successfully for decades. It just works! It's time we brought the truth and the tools necessary to have tremendous healings in everyone's life to the masses. May we all continue to learn the best ways of working with this amazing creation we call the human body.

CHAPTER 1

Every Parent A Chiropractor

I remember as a little kid, my mom used to lay me on the floor facedown and "pop" my back, starting low and going up my spine. It felt great! And I would get out of her hair, run outside and go play for many more hours.

Hint: Want more free time to do what you need to do? Adjust your kids!

I asked Mom how she learned to adjust and she said, "I just always knew." No one ever taught her. Her dad would lie on the floor and ask her to pop his back, and she would just do it as a child.

Hint: If a child can adjust, so can you.

Chiropractors, osteopaths and doctors of physical therapy should have regular classes teaching parents how to adjust their children just like we teach CPR classes to the masses. Until that miracle happens, lay your child face down on the floor. Put your palms down on each side of their spine with your fingers facing away from the middle of their body. Using your thumbs, gently push down and a little up. Lightly work your way up the back one bone at a time until you get to the top of the shoulders or the lower neck. You may or may not hear a "pop." It's okay if it does or doesn't; the pop is not the goal. We're just looking for bones and joints to move and not be stuck. Remember, practice makes perfect, and the more you do it, eventually you'll get a feel for the natural movement of the human body.

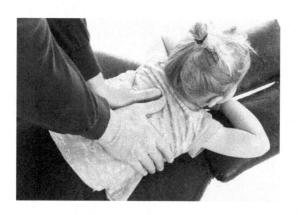

Leave their neck and pelvis alone for now. However, if you hear a pop or feel some shifting while you're checking the mid back, odds are high they'll have a misalignment in their neck or low back as well, and they'll need to be assessed thoroughly by a health care professional.

You may ask, "How often should I check my kids?". This should be done if you ever see or hear from a teacher that your child has taken a fall, which means we're talking about every child. If we're just talking about general maintenance checkups, then the answer is a question: "How long do you want to wait before you find a potentially misaligned vertebrae that is quietly pinching a nerve that you weren't aware they had?" Follow my protocol including my S.E.T. Program outlined in this book, and I guarantee that the number of misaligned vertebrae will decrease as you get comfortable working with your own body and your child's. I check my three-year-old child at least every other day to once per week. I do my S.E.T Program every day because I'm still working on my own correction of an 18mm deficit and I don't want any new misalignments that I might have gotten that day to potentially diminish any level of my health in any way. The traction part of my S.E.T Program is easiest to do daily to three times per week just before I go to bed since I'm already lying down. You'll learn this protocol in the next few chapters.

"How early should I start checking my kids?" I palpated my daughter Presley almost every day to every other day when she was first born. I noticed she started getting locked up in her upper back between her shoulders after about her first month of being handled, nursing, and sleeping in different situations. This continued to be a focal point of mine, so I checked it weekly. Sometimes she needed it and other times not. When she became a toddler and started walking, that spot was still a concern, so I made sure to keep it mobile each time I picked her up.

From the front, I would place one hand under each of her armpits, and my fingertips would fit just perfectly around her chest on each side of her upper back. I would give a little squeeze and a quick gentle acceleration as I lifted her up off the floor. Ninety percent of the time it would release and mobilize, sometimes with multiple pops. She would laugh and giggle and we would share a big hug with the "uppies."

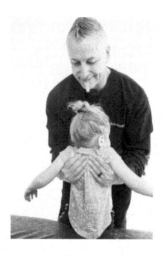

I know it's hard to remember all your trips and falls as a kid. We were all wild, crazy, and fearless! Surely there are a few falls that stick out very clearly in your mind. Odds are you never saw a professional to check and see if you messed something up in your back or neck. Well guess what, if you never did, it's probably still in there! The damage you did when you fell tore the muscle and/or ligament. Ligaments hold your bones in place. There's a one hundred percent chance that you knocked a vertebra out of place. Scar tissue begins forming in the first twelve hours and like a spiderweb, it can glue that vertebrae quickly into a misaligned position. Now it has the potential to start putting pressure on and hurting other structures around it like the delicate soft nerves that are vital to maintaining a healthy-functioning body.

Your parents should have been your first line of defense. After every fall and using the procedure I described above, they should have laid you on the floor and checked to see if anything got stuck or misaligned. Instead, they only checked what they were taught to look for as kids by their parents, generation after generation after generation, and that was to see if there were any broken bones or bleeding. They were never taught to check for mal-positioned joints or to take you to a professional who knew how to find them.

Instead, if there was a question of a possible break, it was a trip to the emergency room for an x-ray. If there was no fracture, then the treatment for a sprain or strain was to brace it and/or refer them to a physical therapist who, in the past, had no clue how to manipulate a misaligned joint. So parents would always do nothing and say "buck up," "walk it off," or "you're fine, just stop crying" or send them to the physical therapist, who would basically only exercise the injured joint and do nothing for a fixated joint.

This primary mechanism of faulty defense means 100 percent of the population has some level of misaligned joints, usually with some level of compensation as well. **This is an epidemic in our society** that is one of the general underlying causes of ill health. Plain and simple: poor structure decreases function and overall health. Thomas Edison said it best, "The doctor of the future will give NO MEDICINE but will interest his patients in the CARE OF THE HUMAN FRAME, diet and in the cause and prevention of disease." Clearly, we are not in the future yet. As a society, we are wallowing in the dregs of treatment protocols, forever learning (and paying) about diseases but never coming to the knowledge of the truth.

We as parents need to be more proactive in the true health of our children, especially during the younger ages where children are growing and physically changing so fast. One small miss of an injured joint will start a chain reaction of compensations that could set your child up for decades of migraines, back or neck pain, or some other acute or chronic disease!

Guess what? You suffered 3,000 falls (for the average teenager) or 5,000 falls if you played sports. Odds are you missed fixing something. You loaded up your backpack with tons of heavy books and carried them all over school, where you sat for twelve years with poor posture. Then you carried it forward and did the same thing in college for however many years you were there. Now, enter the age of technology, and everybody's heads are hanging down and buried in their electronics.

Have you ever heard of a "micro-tear?" Micro-tears can have the same injuries and residuals as a car wreck, only they happen slowly over a longer period of time. For example, looking down while reading a schoolbook, texting on your phone, or staring into a computer screen with your head forward for prolonged periods of time.

Unless you grew up in an ideal world where you had body work (from your parents or a professional) after every single tumble, you've got three strikes against you, and you are out in more ways than you know or can sense. Don't pass down the torch of tradition and make the same mistakes most of our parents made. If you're seeing a doctor who resets joints, have them teach you some simple skills to check your child. Just ask. If they are uncomfortable with that, then you need to find a better practitioner because they are being ruled by money, fear, or lack of education.

I know this book title includes "Avoid Seeing a

Chiropractor," but if you never have or you are not currently seeing a joint setter, then you have not had enough body work to fix your current issues and need some guidance and teachings that this book will surely miss.

Just remember, everyone in this world has the gift of touch. Unless you have HSAN (Hereditary Sensory Autonomic Neuropathy), we can all feel things with our hands and fingers. If you went blind today, I guarantee you still would have the ability to develop the "fine sensitivity" of touch and be able to differentiate between two tiny small bumps while learning how to read brail with practice.

Doing the procedure above may feel a bit awkward at first. You love your child and want what is best for them. I have confidence in you that you will use the right amount of caution and care not to drive their backbone through their chest and into the basement of your house. Kids are tough and you're not going to hurt them. It's a great bonding experience for all involved, and you'll be surprised when they start coming back and asking you to do it again. That's building trust in a family setting and not being ruled by fear anymore.

VISUALIZATION: Imagine a world where every parent is a skilled screener for every bump, bruise and trauma experienced along the way of childhood growth, development, fun, and exploration.

CHAPTER 2

Facts & Fiction

The Knuckle-Cracker

We've all heard, "Don't pop your knuckles, you'll get arthritis" from some queezzer out there. (Queezzer is just a term I created for someone who is uneducated in a matter and doesn't know the truth but speaks as if they do.) For those who cringe at the sound of popping joints, we have an instrument called an "Activator" that just gently taps your bones back into place and makes a small clicking sound. Although this technique is very slow at structural correction, it does have a solid research background for manipulation of a joint. So no excuses not to move forward and visit a joint setter, chiropractor, osteopath or doctor of physical therapy.

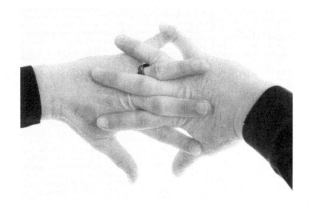

The truth is in knuckle-cracking research: An MD and winner of the Ig Nobel Prize in Medicine, Dr. Donald Unger popped the fingers on his left hand twice a day and not the knuckles on his right—for fifty years! That's cracking at least 36,500 times! X-rays showed no correlation with arthritis. There have also been several other studies, and all had the same results. There is no cause or connection to arthritis in the hands or anywhere else in the body, for that matter. Therefore, be like the concert pianist who mobilizes and clears his fingers before tickling those ivories. Keeping ALL the joints of the body unstuck and moving fully is one of the healthiest practices you can have. Remember, if you're moving, your alive! If you're not moving, then you're dead! That goes for every joint in your body. Now you just need to learn HOW to work with your own body, and that, my friends, is the focus of this book.

Here is the link to the article in the Scientific American journal regarding knuckle-cracking by Dr. Unger.

https://www.scientificamerican.com/article/crack-research/

Bone is Dynamic!

Bone has a remarkable feature in that throughout your entire life, it has the ability to lay down more bone or take it up according to the forces that are applied to it. What this means is your bones are constantly changing. One of the rare characteristics about bone, out of all the cells in your body that heal, is that you can break a bone and it can heal back stronger than it was before. When bones get thin, it's called osteoporosis. Tens of millions of Americans suffer from this, mostly because they don't eat right or get counter pressure or resistance by not exercising enough. When your bones lay down more bone around the joint due to injury and misalignment, it's called degenerative arthritis.

The results of degenerative arthritis are bone spurs and, in the spine, they can grow so large that they pinch nerves and cause a whole other plethora of symptoms and ill health. The problem with this is that in advanced stages when there is no curve in your neck and excessive forward head posture, it will also turn your flexible ligaments and calcify them into bone.

You also must be aware of (and fight against) this epidemic of forward head posture. Every 10mm your head goes out in front of your body while you look down at your phone or computer increases the pressure on your upper back and neck multiplied times two. So the average poor posture texting, about 80mm (3 inches) would equal a 160-pound sack of dog food at the lower neck spinal level. That is enough force to accelerate degenerative arthritis and give you a bone spur in your twenties and thirties! Do you really want that kind of permanent damage?

9.8mS² (Gravity)

There is a force at the core of the Earth that keeps our feet planted on solid ground so we don't go flying off into space, yet pulls downward just enough to drag astronauts, rocks, aliens, and any other flying thing down to the ground at almost ten meters per second squared. It is a force that eventually wins and will put you six feet under the dirt. Let me just say, I have a love-hate relationship with this thing called gravity.

LOVE: I've logged thirty-eight skydives free falling at $9.8mS^2$ or about 120mph, two bungee jumps (one forward, one backwards), seven paraglides floating for hours on the wind at the mountains' crest, and two parasails being pulled behind a boat.

HATE: I'm tired of everything I touch ending up on the floor. Laundry, papers, keys, pacifiers, etc.—you get what I mean. Gravity is a constant force pushing down on your head, and there is nothing you can do about it. It's a never-ending fight throughout life and if you give up, you and other people will notice. You might as well be carrying your head around in your hands!

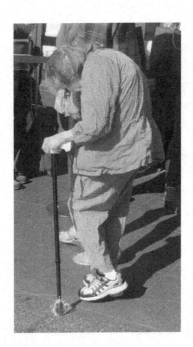

Who wants to stop fighting against gravity and end up like this!

We are all born rounded because we had to curl up like a basketball in our mom's belly. The pinnacle and most important transformation of a rounded curve into the erect human spine is the neck. It begins to form first when you are an infant lying on your stomach and you lift your head up to look around. It continues to form when you begin crawling with your head up and completes its creation upon standing, where it settles into place, hopefully with the head positioned in the center of the shoulders and symmetrically between the chest and back.

Any one of these stages can have developmental problems introduced that will cause the curve of the neck to form improperly, from falls, hits, poor handling, and drops to falling asleep in awkward positions in car seats and on couches. Did I say "drops?" Yes, I did. One research study showed 50 percent of the population are dropped on their head during the first year of life. I was probably one of them, and most go unreported by babysitters.

Remember that, coupled with 3,000 falls for the average teenager, the odds are your neck is so jacked up that by the time you are twenty to thirty years old, you probably have fairly regular headaches or some other warning sign like your hands falling asleep at night, chronic stiff shoulders, etc. Either way, the most important symptom is NO SYMPTOM AT ALL. Like cancer, this problem of a malformed curve of your neck will cause misalignments of the vertebrae which in turn pinch vital nerves and cut off blood flow that control organs and will brew and fester unnoticed for decades, slowly eating away at the core of your health from the inside out. Cavities in teeth don't form overnight and neither does the onset of chronic neck pain unless it came from a specific acute injury.

This curve MUST be restored to its original healthy position in order to avoid seeing a chiropractor extensively. It's as easy as lying on your back with a pool noodle under your neck and doing exercises reverting back and mimicking when you were first placed on your stomach and began lifting your head. The details are explained later in this book under the S.E.T. Program.

The amazing effects of anti- or no gravity is witnessed by NASA's recent study of twins. The astronaut Scott Kelly was sent up to live in space for a full year away from his twin brother Mark. When he returned, they found out he grew two inches taller than his brother, who remained here on Earth! I deduct from the studies that most of the growth was fluid increasing in the discs and joints of the body, not the actual bones growing longer like a giraffe. His bones actually got thinner. A sliver of these results can be measured in each and every one of us. We are all taller in the morning when we wake up from a night of lying down. However, as gravity starts in when we stand, we lose half an inch of height in the first hour we are awake and standing upright and another quarter of an inch throughout the rest of the day.

This is a great spot to pitch bringing back anti-gravity boots! Nowadays we have inversion tables. Everyone should be actively engaged in some sort of inversion protocol (stretch, exercise, or traction). Being upside down fills the discs in between the vertebrae of the spine with essential fluids in order to maintain healthy joints. It also separates compressions caused by arthritis and misalignments. Plus, it makes you taller!

(HINT: If you don't have room for an inversion table, then simply lie face down and hang off the end of your bed, the arm of your couch or a therapy ball from the waist down. You can also use the Roman chair in the gym. It may be necessary to have your partner hold your feet to get the full effect so you don't drop on your head again.)

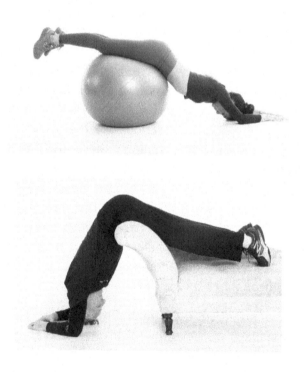

Body Posture

Remember when your mom used to tell you, "Sit up straight!" Well, turns out she was right. Now more than ever, with the introduction of the electronic age in our lives, we must fight every minute of every hour of every workday to rise above the poor aftereffects created by computers that just sit on desk tops. They are literally over two feet out of alignment from our natural body posture, causing us to slump and lean our way into poor health. Most ergonomic charts show that proper computer screen height places the eyes at the top of the screen level. I attest this is absolutely incorrect! The eyes should be at the level of the middle of the screen, and now with the epidemic of forward head posture and loss of the cervical curve, the screen should be placed even higher above the eyes, forcing the head back and the user to be looking up most of the time to aid in proper spinal correction. All cell phone use should be with the phone held up high at eye level. Period. Anything less feeds poor health.

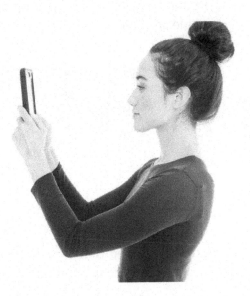

My dad, Staten Sr., is most famous for helping to build the original Batmobile and the Munster's cars from the TV shows. He also went on to work with Gene Winfield to create a few more master custom cars before branching out on his own and creating twenty-five more amazing one-of-a-kind handmade cars. One of his creations is this beautiful Jaguar XJ220 replica modeled after the XJ220 prototype that Jaguar never built. The only people who seem to notice me driving this car around anymore are those who attend car shows where I have it parked. As I pass by any street corner or waiting line (a bus stop, for example), I see 90 percent of the people holding their phones at waist level with their head hanging over the front of their body looking straight down to the ground. Years and decades of this behavior will lead to tremendous ill health that has such a variable negative effect, it can't begin to be measured across a given population. They are missing so much beauty in the environment around them, not to mention that they will never look up and get to enjoy my dad's incredible creation!

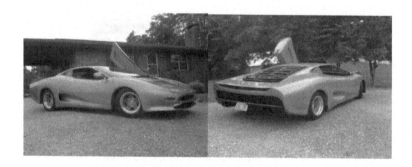

I am shocked and stunned that even in this day and age of advancements and technology, somebody (leading in the fitness industry) just put out a new piece of exercise equipment (one elliptical and one stationary bike machine) that is so biomechanically incorrect, it will strengthen your body and reinforce it in a hunched over, forward posture that is completely counter effective to training the body in an upright position with overall proper alignment. (Beware when you try to purchase online or go into your local gym! You're better off not using the arm handles at all, especially on the ellipticals.)

Us and Them

This is why chiropractic and joint setting is not so common or accepted in the world today. The American Medical Association (AMA) was established in 1847 and fifty-one years later, in 1895 when chiropractic was born, the AMA was very well organized and regulating all medical matters. It's very simple. The AMA said, "Join us." Chiropractors said, "Screw you, we're going to do our own thing!" The AMA (Goliath) then said, "We're going to have you thrown into jail for practicing without a "medical" license. And they did! Not only that, but if you were a medical doctor who referred your patient to a chiropractor, you would lose your medical license. We did establish our own regulatory board, but since 1895 the AMA has put out negative propaganda against chiropractors, which continues today on all social media outlets. Most osteopaths (MDs) were even encouraged not to adjust their patients, but to become general practice pill pushers. I know this because I retrained many osteopaths how to adjust when they desired to pick up the manipulating art again. This fact was proven in a court of law finally in 1985, when chiropractors won the lawsuit against the AMA for its decades of harassments.

It took chiropractors twelve years of jailing to organize the Universal Chiropractors Association (UCA), established at the Palmer School of Chiropractic in 1906, to thwart efforts by organized medicine (MDs) to jail DCs. No wonder there's a huge, deep ravine filled with so much animosity separating the two professions. We just got started off on the wrong foot. In the words of Jack Nicholson, "Why can't we all just get along!"

Since then, chiropractors and their affiliates have spent most of our profession's money fighting to prove we're a legitimate entity worthy of the table scraps thrown out by government law and private insurance companies' colossal financial wealth of "force pay." There's a saying in chiropractic: "We eat our young." Those new in the profession who fought tooth and nail to survive and make a buck were usually devoured by some overprotective contract in favor of their DC boss that stripped them of any chance of success while working, especially taken when they left the "associate doctor" position. Most of those who found the cash train hoarded their money selfishly, which meant there were never enough funds put into public education and awareness to teach you (like dentistry has done) that EVERYONE should visit a chiropractor at least every six months. Instead, after 123 years of just trying to keep our heads afloat and stay the inevitable endless abyss, less than 10 percent of the population utilizes our services and that, my friends, is just whacked.

I know of a "dental park" complex consisting of three buildings, each three stories high, and all filled with mainly dentists and their supporting businesses, and they are all packed with patients. The chiropractic representation should be no different. Ninety percent of the population need us but just simply aren't aware yet that they do.

In God's infinite wisdom, I have worked and been accepted by both sides of the fence. I was in the hospital setting for three years while I completed my pre-med. I worked my way up in a small community hospital in Tomball, Texas and went from an admission coordinator to running all the nurses' stations throughout the facility. I even transferred to a bigger hospital in downtown Houston while I was searching for my specialty in medicine. Not feeling the hospital vibe and turning toward private practices, I bounced from veterinary medicine to in-home care services and eventually ended up working for a chiropractor as an exam clinician.

The blood, the gore, the sickness, the mistakes, the bickering between doctors and nurses as to who "knows what's best" for the patients were all drivers for me to keep looking outside of the hospital field. Bagging bodies of patients with whom I had become friendly within the chemo/oncology field was no joy ride either. Neither was working in the ER and seeing the human body blown up, shot up, cut up, or mangled. It hurt my empathetic soul too much. I left with super high admiration for those in the field who could care for the population in that way. It just wasn't me.

I didn't find the right path until I worked as a chiropractic assistant. I was conducting my own little research study while doing exams and x-rays of all the new patients and then thirty days later doing a re-exam and going over their findings with them.

EVERY single patient got better! Their demeanor was happier, their energy was boosted, and the reason why was right there in front of me in black and white. A lot of the initial tests that were given were positive at first, and now they were negative. Their range of motion increased dramatically. Their pain was diminished, and they were by far a better person overall than the first day they walked into my exam room. I was shocked and amazed as the re-exams of betterment kept coming, one after the other after another. I thought, "What is this wonderful healing art that I have stumbled across?" I say it was "only by chance" that I got that job, but the reality is that private practice medical doctors wouldn't hire me because I didn't have experience drawing blood. I just wanted a job in a doctor's office outside of the hospital setting. The process of elimination was implemented appropriately, and I now found a new directive in life. I wanted to be a chiropractic doctor instead of a medical doctor. (Although I wasn't aware of osteopaths at this time. Had I, my outcome might be quite different.)

Later in practice, I did become one of the team physicians for the pro soccer team the Salt Lake Real. Although the players loved me, there was quite the conflict and competition between me and the physical therapist. I'd like to think this is easing up as society gets older and hopefully wiser.

I AM what I am. Regardless of any social title, I am a true gifted healer. A healer of the mind, soul, body, family, community, entities, governments, countries, and worlds, if so called. My best mediums are mastered through touch, music, and the spoken word.

Stemming from a vision I had five years ago, I am motivated and vow to do my best to heal what may seem irreconcilable differences between my two professions. Therefore, I was inspired from above to create the "Ad-Man Census," a worldwide adjustment/manipulation census to get ALL the professions that adjust the spine working together on a single cause. Since there is no accurate data, let's just simply count how many people receive the benefit of manipulations around the world and use that data to compare the health of each community.

(HINT: For more detail on this and my other journeys, read my next book, *Transitions: Coping in a Cracked-Up World*) release date TBD.

Once You Go, You Always Go

I've also heard that once you go to the dentist, you have to go for the rest of your life. Good spinal health is no different. How much more vital is the spine and the nerve system that controls everything in your body compared to a pretty smile. Every person on the planet deserves, at bare minimum, a healthy spine to give them the most optimum human experience possible in life. Everything works better when your engine is firing on all cylinders. So, like dentistry, go to a joint setter a minimum every six months. Remember, it's best to go when you feel good. Waiting until your problems become symptomatic with tons of pain and muscle spasms removes you from having an enjoyable experience with your professional. Who wants to be poked at when you're already in so much pain? It's just easier to fix problems when you don't hurt.

Unfortunately, most people wait to see a chiropractor until they're 20 or 30 years into a twisted-up spine. That's like going to the dentist for the first time as an adult and him telling you that you need six cavities filled, four of which need root canals, one tooth needs to be pulled, and you'll need braces on your teeth after all that work. It takes much more time to fix issues that have been in there festering for years than it does to maintain your body with a checkup every six months. Hopefully someday our society will flip the switch in their head and accept the comparison as second nature, so that when you ask anyone, "How often are you supposed to see the chiropractor," they respond with the same answer as if you'd said, "How often are you supposed to see a dentist?" Every six months at first, and then after your issues are corrected/fixed you should have a checkup a minimum of every six months thereafter.

Until that day, chiropractors will just be minimally known as "back pain" doctors and a last-ditch chance modality to try if the medical field failed to fix the problem. This is because drugs, surgery, and exercises from a physical therapist are engrained and programmed as the only first-choice options for soft tissue injuries. We all know where that has led our society. We've got the most expensive healthcare system with the worst level of overall health per capita and the largest opioid addiction in history, and we wonder why our homeless encampments are growing at such an alarming rate. I've heard it said that the chiropractic profession is still 40 years behind the dental industry in its campaign to change the public's perception of spinal health as the core focus of attention and initial treatment.

Oh, Now I Get It!

It's not rocket science, people. The template is already laid out before you and you just need to connect the dots in your head. Simply apply the protocol of dentistry to chiropractic (or any manipulating profession, like osteopathic.) Dentistry begins when you have teeth. Chiropractic begins when you have a spine. Once you have teeth, you should visit the dentist every six months for a checkup. For chiropractic, especially for children, because you can catch so many things and fix them easier than if you wait 10 or 20 years before your first visit. EVERY child's spine should be checked at birth for any trauma introduced from the birthing process. This is NEVER done in a medical setting. The best you'll get is an APGAR test one minute after birth.

APGAR stands for "Appearance" of skin color, "Pulse" rate of the heart, "Grimace" like irritability or crying, "Activity" of movement or reflex to stimulation, and how fast are their "Respirations" or breaths. Of course, they count fingers and toes, but that's the extent of the exam. Trauma to the newborn can be introduced at any stage of birth, starting with the mom's crooked pelvis. Most expectant mothers never had chiropractic care growing up and therefore have a high incidence of rotated or misaligned pelvis. This makes it easy for the baby to get hung up on the mom's pelvis, which causes fetal stress, resulting in a "failure to progress" situation that inevitably leads to an emergency C-section. I just saw in the news recently that C-sections are now being done at a staggering rate of over 32 percent of all births!

Trauma is introduced when the baby's head is halfway down the birth canal, at which point the baby gets pulled backwards out by the feet, causing traction while twisting the head and neck severely. Other traumas can come from improper handling—like the old cliché says, "I'm late for my tee off!"—as the doctor begins tugging or pulling on the baby excessively, or even worse, introduces a tool-like clamping forceps or a "screw in the top" skull cap for vacuum suction. Also, expectant mothers are regularly induced (by recommendation or by selfish choice) and force the baby to exit before they are ready to engage this colossal first challenge of life. Again, all the more reason to allow joint setting to simply correct a misaligned baby or mother's pelvis as soon as possible! Even during pregnancy, joint setting has monumental positive impact to both parties.

CHAPTER 3

The Simple Start

General Care in the Morning (Your First Self-Adjustment)

Good morning! You are already lying down in your bed, hopefully from a well-rested sleep. It's so easy to start your first yoga stretch of the day right there. Remember, you grew one inch last night. You are at your tallest when you first wake up. Let's use that extra height to mobilize any stuck joints acquired from a possibly funky mosh pit of tag team acrobatic sleeping. Stretching is the first stage of self-adjusting. We will start off doing the reclined spinal twist. Lie down on your left side with your legs straight, bend your right knee and lock your right foot behind your left knee. Put your left hand on your right knee and turn your upper body and head in the opposite direction to the right while reaching out with your right hand to the right like your body is a wet hand towel being wrung out. Now put a little downward pressure on your right knee, pressing it gently toward the floor, and let the cavitation's begin. Breath slowly and deeply and count to twenty. Repeat for the opposite side.

(Hint: This is a perfect moment to have a spiritual connection with your Higher Power by giving thanks for the day and contemplating your day's events.)

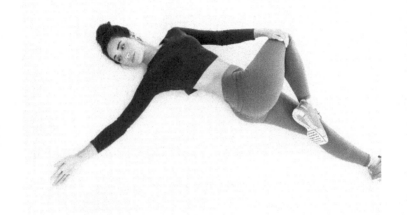

A cavitation (or "pop" sound) during a stretch is NOT an adjustment. It is simply an opening of the joint and a release of carbon dioxide, like when you open a soda can. An adjustment or manipulation is when you put your finger right on the bone and push it to move it. That maneuver may or may not cause a cavitation. It doesn't matter and should not be the goal. Here, we are doing just a general stretch of the pelvis, specifically the SI (sacroiliac) joint, and if something opens quickly, it may release some air.

Next, keep that same position, but now modify it and pretend you are the "walk/don't walk" guy in the lit crosswalk sign. Take your right leg and straighten it out to the left as far as you can, this time reaching underneath your leg and grabbing the ankle if you can reach it with your left hand. Keep the rest of the upper body in the same position to the right as the previous stretch. This one focuses more on the connective muscles and ligaments of the legs and (low back) torso to the pelvis. Repeat for the opposite side. (Namaste: I see the light in you, and it is good.)

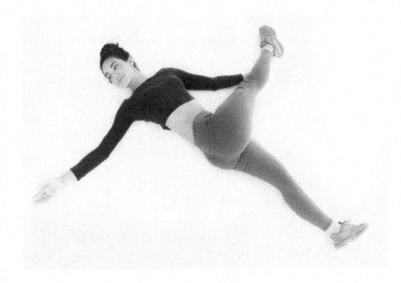

The second stage of self-manipulation is an exercise in each of these positions. Simply come out of the position slightly, and with a pumping action, go back into the stretched position. Repeat this bouncing action for 10 repetitions.

I know this is starting to sound like an exaggerated game of Twister, but in this basic position you can now introduce a contact point and a thrust to adjust your own lower back. For example, in the second position we just did, with your right leg stretched straight out to the left, take your right hand and make a fist with your thumb on the outside/topside of your fist and sticking up a bit and your first finger/knuckle pushed out a little from the rest. Use the pad of your thumb and the knuckle of your first finger for precise contact. Contact as high as you can reach up the spine to the side of a vertebra in your lower back, not directly on the middle of the spine but about

27

half an inch (one thumb thickness) off-center on the "up" side closest toward the ceiling. Simultaneously, gently push in with your thumb while you swing your right leg a little more to the left and down. Move about an inch down to the next vertebra and repeat the maneuver until you reach the pelvis. (If you feel any sharp pain, go visit your joint setting specialist or health care professional. Your spine is possibly too far damaged to handle a self-manipulation regimen.)

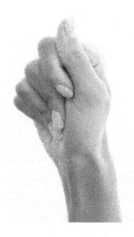
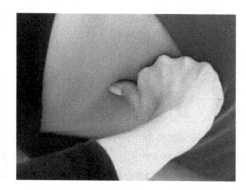

(HINT: For better leverage, go to the edge of your mattress and in the first position, lock the heel of your top foot into the side of the mattress for counter pressure against your fist/thumb.)

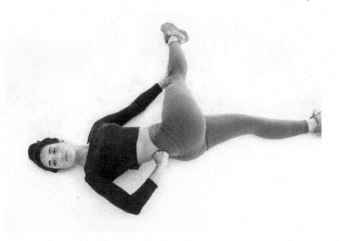

Yes, No, I Don't Know

There are three basic movements in the neck that will stretch almost every muscle in your neck and shoulder region and get you ready for a self-manipulation procedure. They are the x, y, and z axis that the head pivots on. "Yes" is Flexion and Extension. (Looking up and looking down.) "No" is right and left Rotation (looking over your shoulders.) "I don't know" is Lateral Flexion or ear toward your shoulders. These three movements can be used as a stretch (that you hold for 20 twenty seconds) and as an exercise (for example, doing three sets of ten repetitions).

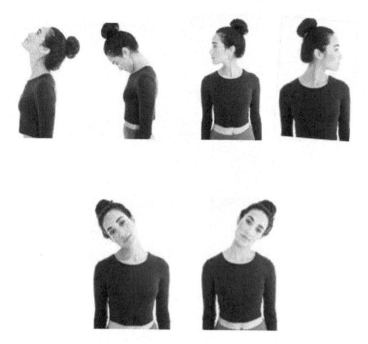

(Hint 1: If you feel no pain during these stretches, you can add a little extra pressure at the end point by putting your hand on your cheek or top of your head while doing each maneuver.)

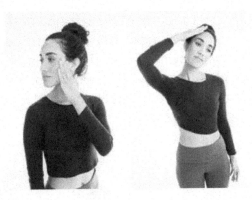

(Hint 2: Do each of these ranges of motion as a "rocking back and forth" exercise through each plane to train the bones in your neck to track in simple directions, especially if you have any old injuries that have reduced your ability to look <u>fully</u> in any direction. Example: If you can't turn your head and look over your shoulder in your blind spot while driving, or if you turn your chin toward your shoulder in rotation <u>naturally without forcing it</u> and it doesn't go 80 degrees and line up with your shoulder, then you are limited in your range and this exercise will benefit you most.)

You should definitely do all three as a stretch while sitting on your bed first thing in the morning, but to self-adjust, the best direction is in the "I don't know" plane of motion.

Here's how: Simply use two or three fingers pointing straight as a stern fulcrum of one hand and put them on the side of the neck/spine. With the opposite hand using three fingers, contact the top of the head on the opposite side and gently push toward the shoulder at the same time. For example, if the right hand/fingers contact the spine, then you will push toward the left shoulder. Simultaneously the left

31

hand/fingers contact the top of the left side of the head and push toward the right shoulder. Start high just below the ear and work your way down one vertebra level or one inch at a time with a gentle push. Repeat for each side. (If you feel any sharp pain, you should stop the maneuver and seek out a professional to assess the dysfunction.)

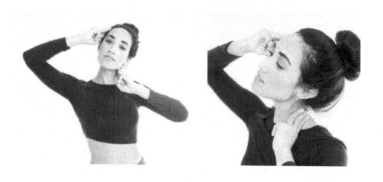

(Hint 1: You can also do this maneuver without contacting the top of the head with your opposite hand and just move your head with your ear going toward the same shoulder that your spinal contact hand is on.)

(Hint 2: Never grab your chin with the palm of your hand and forcefully push up to the right or the left! This creates hypermobile segments that move too much and make it extremely difficult for an experienced joint setter to correct and stabilize.)

Your Weakest Link

A chain is only as strong as its weakest link. Link together two bulldozers with a chain and have them pull it until it snaps.

The link that broke is the one with the most imperfections in its creation. Your muscles and ligaments have undergone some tremendous negative forces over the years. There are hundreds and thousands of micro- and macro-tears everywhere and in so many different directions.

Your injured joints are your weakest link in your spine. If they are not treated with joint manipulation, they will follow the three characteristics of scar tissue. 1) Scar tissue is like a spiderweb only with fibers completely unorganized and all over the place in different directions. 2) It has more pain fibers in it than any regular tissue and therefore hurts more. 3) It shrinks. Especially when tension on it is laxed or it's cold. This shrinking takes place at night when you sleep so you wake up stiff in the morning or during the winter months when temperatures reduce. This is why all the old folks move down south when they retire, so they can be in the warmer climate states. It doesn't flare up, shrink and fire off the scar tissue surrounding their joints as much.

My dad is a prime example of this, having moved down to Las Vegas from Seattle. After three failed low back surgeries and living in severe pain every single day, relying on extreme doses of morphine to get by, he now feels like he's nineteen years old again and wants to buy a dirt bike because his back isn't flaring up like it was in the cold Seattle weather.

Microscopically, joint manipulation makes the spiderweb line up along the regular growth pattern of the muscles and ligaments. Therefore, if the scar tissue does shrink, it doesn't pull the joint out of alignment. It just gets tight. Manually thrusting into a joint is also proven to break up pain fibers and reduce the sensations that pain gives out in an area. After the joints have been "unstuck," the most important regimen to keep the total body moving properly is gentle, easy yoga. However, if you do not go through some manipulation regimen prior to yoga, you are creating compensations that will eventually surface.

I was the chiropractor for Ringling Bros. and Barnum & Bailey Circus when they came through town. I would adjust most all of the performers including the elephants, big cats, dogs, and horses. (Yes, they have spines too and are under tremendous stress from their continued unique activities.) I've also been known to adjust the "Bear/Cougar dogs" for the Washington Department of Fish and Wildlife, as well as the bomb squad dogs and the horses for the Seattle police department. Occasionally I've adjusted a snake, a lizard, a rabbit, and even a fish that was bent when the pond was struck by lightning!

One thing I noticed is that the acrobats in the circus were the healthiest athletes I've ever seen in any given population of sports. They constantly worked with their bodies every single day, pushing it to its extremes. The body adapted and remained flexible and required hardly any manipulation on my part.

The Upper Back Self-Adjusting

This next maneuver is for your middle and upper back. This is the most difficult part of the spine to self-adjust because it's almost impossible to reach with your own hands, therefore it's best to use fulcrums or secondary aids. The best device I have found to actively assist in self-mobilizing the upper back is called the "Still Point Inducer." I highly recommend you purchase one.

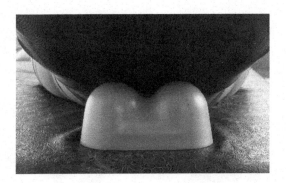

Place the fulcrum on the edge of your bed mattress. Lie on your back with the fulcrum positioned at the uppermost part of the upper back just below the neck. Raise both arms above your head and repeatedly and forcefully thrust them up and down toward the ceiling and the floor. After several times, move the fulcrum down one inch (or scoot your body up) to the next vertebra level and repeat. Continue this maneuver down the spine until you get to the top of the low back. You'll feel where the spine curves and the fulcrum no longer become beneficial and loses its effectiveness.

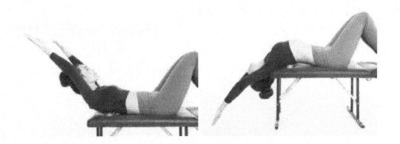

(Hint: Alternate thrusting your arms at angles more off to the sides instead of straight over your head.)

The following stretches can be done prior to prep the area or to help keep the upper back mobile after it has gone through a manipulative procedure to unlock it. I call this first one the Modified Extended Child Pose.

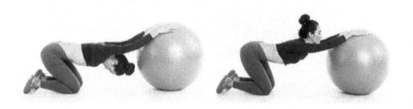

Get down on your hands and knees and rest your forearms on a couch or a therapy ball. The maneuver is done two separate ways. In both, push your chest down toward the floor. Do this once with your head up and once with your head down. This will isolate the upper back between the shoulder blades to keep it movable.

Next is the Modified Extended Child Pose Reach Through. Get down on your hands and knees. Take your right arm and dive it under your left arm with your palm facing upward as you roll down upon your right shoulder blade. Feel free to rock around at different angles to get the force into the desired area in the upper back. Repeat for the opposite side.

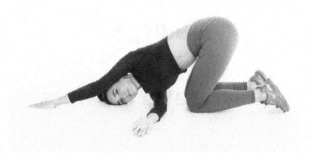

(Hint: This is also a good time to do the standard "Spinal Twist" in yoga.)

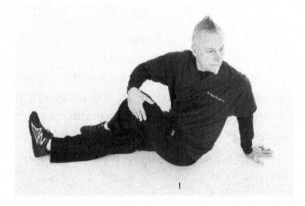

CHAPTER 4

The Meat & Potatoes

Your Own Personal S.E.T. Program

This S.E.T. Program was created after 30 years of working on musicians and needing to give them the best possible treatment information that would last the longest, since I wouldn't see them for at least another six months to a year when they came through town again on their next tour. I had to assess them quickly and thoroughly and write my findings down on a paper that they could take with them to review and follow easily. By committing to my program, they were definitely better or at least not worse the next time I saw them. The program had actually worked! I tweaked it a few times over the years and it proves itself every time. You DO my program, you WILL get better!

Your S.E.T. Program

<u>Stretching / Exercise / Traction</u>

Stretching: Making tight muscles <u>longer</u> with sustained tension. (Hold for 20 seconds)

Exercise: Making muscles <u>shorter</u> with repeated resistance (3 Sets of "fatigue" reps)

Traction: Making ligaments <u>smarter</u>. "Braces on Teeth". (Hold up to 20 min./day)

<u>STRETCHES (Daily)</u>

- Neck (Yes, No, I Don't Know)
- Chest (Hold Thru Doorway)
- Right Hamstring
- Left Hamstring
- Right Quad
- Left Quad
- Therapy Ball: Lie on Back
- Foam Roll _____
- Other:_____

<u>EXERCISES (3x/Week)</u>

- Cervical Extension (Look Up)
- Cervical Translation (Push Chin In)
- Right Hamstring (Leg Curls)
- Left Hamstring (Leg Curls)
- Right Quad (Leg Extensions)
- Left Quad (Leg Extensions)
- Robot 10x a Day
- Seated Rows, Lat Pull Downs
- Other:_____

TRACTION (Daily)

◻ **Cervical:** Lie on back on bed with head hanging over the edge of the mattress. (Correcting _____mm.) Neck roll at _____ for 3 months, then at _____ for 3 months. (Add 1 minute per night until 20 min. max.)

◻ **Thoracic:** Lie on your right / left side with a support roll at _____.

◻ **Lumbar:** Lie on your right / left side with a support roll at _____.

◻ **Pelvic:** Use "Pelvic Blocks"/ rolled bath towels daily for _____ months. Lie on back on bed or floor. Right Side: High/Low; Left Side: High/Low. (I am correcting Short R / L _____mm.)

*Absolutely: NO RUNNING, JUMPING, SQUATS, LUNGES or SITTING CROSS-LEGGED

*NO wallets in back pockets and NO heavy purses on one shoulder!

*All upper body exercises with weights are to be done sitting down or lying down!

*All stretches and exercises are to be done in 3 different angles like a clock. (Ex: 10, 12, and 2 o'clock)

P.O. Box 1433
Mercer Island, WA 98040

Email:
Rockndoc4@yahoo.com

FB: DrStaten C Medsker

FB Official Fan Page:
CEOdrStatenMedsker

From all of life's traumas you have created an imbalance in your body, mostly in the pelvis and neck. The pelvis is not that complicated when trying to create general healing. It only has three major joints, and they work together to keep your foundation stable and walking. Under a large microscope, or rather in the overall big picture, when you fell, you either pushed the pelvis to the right or to the left when you hit the ground on your butt. Which means it went forward or backwards on any given side. A level of torque was introduced that will pull one leg up and push the other leg down. All we have to do is determine the accurate short side.

This is where the "leg check" comes in. You can get an idea for yourself if you lie on your back and put your feet together, look down and see which heel of your shoe is longer than the other. You can also check the wear on the bottom soles of your old shoes. The shoe with the most wear on the heals is usually the longer leg. Best, though, is to have another person do the measuring (especially better is a skilled professional for accuracy). I measure in millimeters.

I have found that the average person can correct most short leg syndromes an average of 2mm a month and return the pelvis back to a normal level on my program.

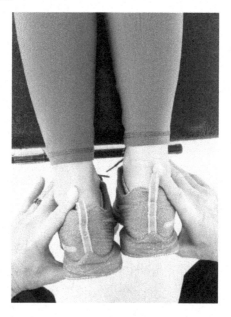

This is where your savings can really weigh in. For example, in a clinical setting, let's say a patient comes to me for care and we measure a 7mm short leg on the right. If I'm going to fix it for the patient and they don't do any work on their own, I can fix 2mm a month if the patient is coming in three times per week. At $50 a visit, that amounts to $600 a month for 3 months, so $1,800 total.

If they're on my S.E.T. program and they do most of the work at home on their own, they only need to come in a minimum of one time per month, (in severe cases you may choose one time per week) thus saving $1,650 and they'll still have the exact same results!

My S.E.T. Program is just like braces on teeth. You do it for a specific amount of time until the correction is accomplished, and then you stop my program and return to your regular symmetrical generic exercise program. (All maintaining proper form and posture, of course.)

Stretches (should be done daily) are designed to make muscles and ligaments longer by holding them at an end range of motion with steady pressure for a good 20 seconds. Exercises (should be done three times per week) contract muscles and make them shorter and are done in three sets of ten repetitions. Traction (should be done daily) makes ligaments and tendons smarter and are sustained stretches (without muscle contraction) that can be held for twenty minutes or longer. **S**tretches, **E**xercises, and **T**raction. This is where I get the acronym for my "S.E.T." Program.

For the sake of uniformity and ease, we are going to assume the person in my example presents with a short **RIGHT** leg. If you have a short left leg, then everything in the next example will be opposite for you. The unilateral (one-sided) stretching (holding for twenty seconds) protocol would be to stretch the **RIGHT** hamstring and the **LEFT** quadricep **ONLY**. The unilateral exercise (three sets of ten) protocol would be to exercise the **LEFT** hamstring and the **RIGHT** quadricep **ONLY**. The most important thing (and my trade secret as to why I get amazing results) when doing these is that they must be done in three different angles in order to be effective.

Arms and legs are round. Muscles are round. So stretch and exercise them round like a clock. For example, there are four muscles in your quad. Instead of doing just the "runner's" stretch that we've all been taught, do one stretch straight on, one stretch with your foot in internal rotation and one stretch in external rotation. The same goes for the hamstring stretches. That way, you stretch all the muscles in the muscle group and get the most effective benefit out of elongating the muscles. If you only stretch one angle, you still have all the other muscles in that group that are left tight, and three tight shorter muscles will retract one long stretched muscle in the same group every time leaving you with negative results.

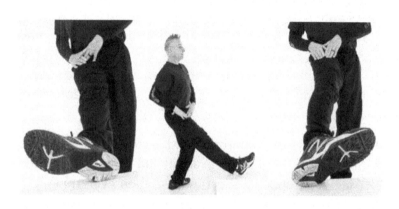

The same concept is carried through with the exercises. You must do three sets. Do one set straight on, one set with your foot in internal rotation and one set with your foot in external rotation. It's this kind of expertise protocol that will assist the traction in making your short leg longer and your long leg shorter.

Traction is the final clincher that solidifies your correction, and you'll find it very soothing and comfortable to do. Purchase a pair of "pelvic blocks" on Amazon for $28.

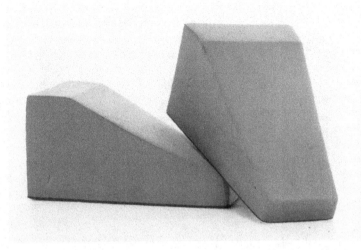

Otherwise, roll up two bath towels or two rolls of paper towels. It takes the average person fifteen to twenty minutes to fall asleep once they lie down in bed. Utilize this time to lie on your blocks. Still utilizing our RIGHT short leg scenario, lie on your back and place one block high on the right pelvis at a 45-degree angle and place the other block low on the left pelvis at a 45-degree angle. (Blocks are pointing toward each other.)

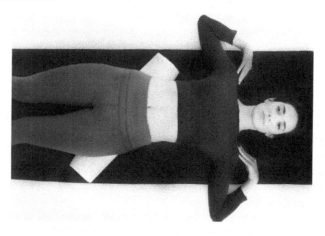

Placement of pelvic blocks if you are short **<u>RIGHT</u>** leg.

When you're about to fall asleep, take the blocks out, put them on your dresser, roll over and fall asleep. It's that simple. This procedure does the exact same thing as a chiropractor lying you on your side and doing a side posture pelvic adjustment. (Like previously stated, if you feel any sharp pain while on the blocks, remove them and consult a joint setting professional.) Otherwise, continue this program and check in with your doctor a minimum of one time per month (although once a week is better) to get an accurate leg measurement to determine that you are still on course for correction. (It's okay and suggested to push the blocks in as far as you can but at your level of comfort.)

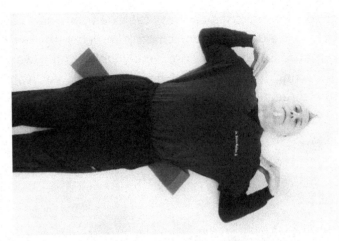

Placement of pelvic blocks if you are short **LEFT** leg.

Finally, cervical/neck protocol for the S.E.T. program. With the introduction of the age of electronics, the average person now has a minimum of 30mm of AWB (Anterior Weight Bearing or forward head posture). This is the equivalent of walking around with a 60-pound sack of potatoes on your head, causing chronic tight neck and shoulder muscles with all the secondary health issues like headaches, migraines, sleeping problems, etc., not to mention that it just looks horrible.

My fail proof stretches, exercises, and traction program will correct a minimum of five millimeters a month of AWB, and it's as simple as taking a two or three inch round fulcrum, a rolled-up hand towel, or cutting about six inches off the end of a pool noodle, and lying down on your back with it placed under your upper back or neck. First, the stretches. Stretches for the neck are the "Yes, No, I don't knows" that were already discussed previously in this book.

Second, the exercises are cervical extensions and cervical translations. Lie on your stomach on your bed with your head off the mattress. Extensions are simply looking up toward the ceiling starting from a neutral position. (Hint: you can also apply the three different angles to this exercise.)

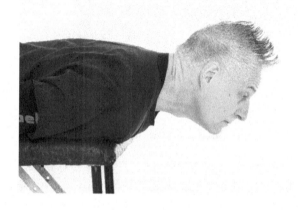

Next are the translations. Start from a neutral position and drive the chin toward the ceiling. This is only a one-inch maneuver. Don't drop your head too far toward the floor upon returning to the neutral position. (Not so flattery but very effective for self-correction.)

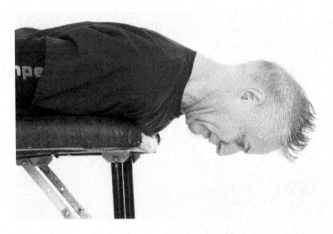

The traction is best done lying on your back on your mattress with your head hanging as far off of the edge of the mattress as possible. For the first three months, the pool noodle is placed at "T2." There are seven vertebrae in your neck. Next below that is a large bump, and on most people, that is T1. Simply place the pool noodle below that bump and let your head traction completely off the end of the mattress. This is to get the head positioned back over the shoulders first.

For the next three months, move the pool noodle to the neck at C6 (just above the large bump). It is imperative that you take your time with this procedure. The goal is to last twenty minutes in this position, but the truth is most people can only last a few minutes when beginning this traction. When it gets uncomfortable, stop the traction, slide back down on your mattress so that your head is supported fully on the bed and then move the pool noodle under the middle of the neck and finish off the rest of the twenty minutes. Gradually add a minute each week, and eventually your neck will adapt to the traction. This maneuver is to restore the curve back into your neck.

(Hint: You can do the cervical traction and the pelvis traction at the same time.)

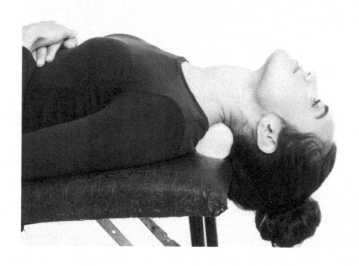

(HINT: Make sure the pool noodle is placed more on the corner edge of the mattress each time you begin the cervical traction, so your head is off of the mattress as far as possible.)

ADDITIONAL STRETCHES AND EXERCISES:

A therapy ball should be your best friend in your program. All stretches and exercises can be done standing, sitting, or lying down. A lot of them can be done using the therapy ball. Outside of the regular S.E.T. Program, the best stretch is just a simple backbend over the ball. Doing this stretch opens the entire body that has been closed off and rounded forward, curling around our books, computers, and social life for decades.

I recommend a daily regimen of stretching the chest. Step into a doorway and place both hands on the side of the door frame. Step through, keeping the head up in extension and opening the chest. Hold for twenty seconds and remember to do at three different angles. Putting the hands low, then medium, and finishing high on the door frame if you can reach it.

Here's one you can have fun with. I call it "the robot."

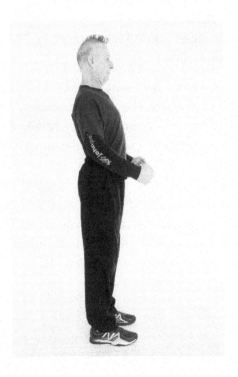

This exercise should be done at least ten times per day. As a reminder, I used to take Post-it notes and write "Robot" on them, then place them throughout my house. On every door as you walk into a new room, on the bathroom mirror, on the fridge, etc. (even on the rearview mirror in my car!). Every time I saw a note, I would do the robot exercise until I changed my posture to fit whatever project I was going into the next room to do.

Stand as upright and erect as you can. Drive your chin backwards into your body. Throw your shoulders back, squeeze your shoulder blades together and push your chest out. Most importantly, stick your butt out! Now finish off with a slight bend in your knees and making sure your feet are shoulder-width apart and facing directly forward without rotating out like a duck.

One of the most frequent conversations I have with patients is the position of the pelvis. So many have been told to tuck their pelvis in or forward, especially by their dance teachers. Although this is great for dancing, it is horrible for the overall function of the pelvis in daily activities. Over 90 percent of my patients had a shallow "sacral base angle" on their x-rays, meaning their pelvis was positioned too far forward. This means 90 percent of you need to STICK YOUR BUTT OUT! Practice makes perfect, and muscle memory wins every time. So, go to it and start the trend!

CHAPTER 5

The Cleanup

Here are a few do's, don'ts and disclaimers. This program WILL change the structure of your skeleton. Like braces on teeth, it is to be done for a finite period of time and then the program should be stopped once you've reached your optimum level of desired correction. This point should be determined between you and your health care professional. You don't want to over-correct and start twisting your body in the opposite direction.

<u>You cannot do this program by yourself</u>. You must have a health care professional who is an expert in accurate leg length measuring and joint setting monitor you through. This is not to replace your chiropractic, osteopathic or physical therapy care, only to enhance it by being proactive and doing more for yourself. Doing this program WILL save you time and money from extensive visits to your joint setting professional. Any health care professional who does not endorse this program by empowering and "teaching the patient to fish" is greedy and selfish and just wants all the money from your extensive visits for themselves.

Absolute don'ts: There should be NO running, jumping, squats, lunges, sitting cross-legged, carrying things in your back pockets (like wallets) and no heavy purses on one shoulder (crossbody straps only). ALL upper body exercises with weights should be done sitting down or lying down to take the load off your crooked pelvis. All stretches and exercises are to be done at three different angles (using your arms and legs twisting around like a clock). All electronics are to be held at eye level (or above) at all times.

A lot of people ask me, "Can I still do my regular exercise routine or run or train for a specific event while on this program?" You can as long as you follow the absolute don'ts listed above. Remember, if you run, it's going to set you back in your correction; therefore, you will have to double up on your blocking and stretches in the program to offset the damage. Remember, if you hammer on a bent nail, the nail bends more. The average most will be on this program is usually between three and six months. Because of the severity, some neck traction candidates will be on the neck traction program for over a year.

As I said, this program is not to replace any treatment program set up by your health care professional, only to enhance it and empower you and educate you to do more for yourself. This is a very general program designed for the masses. Your health care professional can tweak and modify it accordingly to your specific needs.

False positives can occur in about 30 percent of the population during leg check measurements and should be ruled out by your health care professional. These are normally caused by a psoas muscle spasm and result in a short leg on the opposite side of the pelvis-proven short leg. I usually clear these out in the first three visits, then we're left with a true depiction of the short side. Hip and knee surgeries can affect the accuracy of the leg length significantly and should be considered by the expert before beginning this program.

Stop this program immediately if you have herniated/bulging disc issues or sharp pain while doing this program.

Like not being able to eat a steak the day after your get the braces on your teeth tightened, it's okay to experience some muscle soreness the day after doing my S.E.T. Program. Let the body catch up to the corrections you are implementing and continue at a pace that is comfortable for you. The amount of correction you do in a day, week, or month is totally up to you and your body's physical and mental ability to handle the change.

CHAPTER 6

Looking For Mr(s) Right!

The first thing I do when I move into a new area is to go into each chiropractor's office and swap adjustments via "professional courtesy". They adjust me and then I reciprocate. Many times, the doctor would excitedly call in his staff and say, "You've got to get adjusted by this guy! He's amazing!" This helps me learn the thoroughness, accuracy, and the level of their touch they provide to their patients. My underlying interest for doing this is that I'm actually looking for a chiropractor for myself whom I can trust with a high level of skill and comfort working with my own body.

I have extensive experience in this, in that I'm fifty-six years old and have moved fifty-four times in my life. I have adjusted and been adjusted by a large pool of practitioners.

The protocol taught to all doctors goes something like this:

1. Take a lengthy and thorough case history

2. Do an extensive examination

3. Order and take tests (like X-rays/MRI/CT, etc.) to confirm findings

4. Begin treatment or refer out

Most times, it took me going to seven or eight offices before I found a doctor I liked. Searching for the right one can be very expensive following the above protocol each time. Without a "professional courtesy", we're talking $180 to $250 a pop just to find out that the doctor is way under par with their skill level. With my "Mobile" Chiropractic business, in the last thirty years I have adjusted over 360,000 individuals, most of them on site at concerts or shows without x-rays. Just simply mobilizing the stuck joints of the body and being careful not to move joints that are not ready to move. When I finished my work, 99.9 percent of them had an amazing "WOW!" experience. You should too.

If a potential patient walked into my clinic and said, "Look, I'm shopping for a chiropractor and I'd like to see if your style/technique of adjusting works for me. I don't want to spend all the upfront cost of exams and x-rays. Can you just adjust me so I can get a sense of your healing touch?" If they don't say, "Lie facedown and let's get started," say, "Thank you" and turn around and walk out the door and move on to the next clinic down the road. If they are confident enough in their abilities, it should be as simple as signing a release and them saying, "Come on back and lie face down!"

(Disclaimer: I'm not telling the doctor to go against state and national protocol rules. I'm saying there is a brief protocol that follows the rules to expedite and qualify the patient for quick treatment.)

Once the doctor has agreed to adjust you, the first question out of your mouth should be, "Do you do leg length measurements?" The accuracy and art of measuring leg length is crucial to monitoring your progress. Again, if they are not skilled in this test, go interview the doctor on the next corner. I'm not talking about just seeing if one leg is shorter than the other leg. Anyone can do that. I'm saying that they need to tell you in millimeters or inches how far off your legs are on each visit. This alone is a mastered skill learned over time.

Just like a professional construction worker who doesn't need to use a tape measure or ruler every time anymore because he's done it a million times and the distance of "one inch" like a caliber is burned into his brain. My internal gauge is 7mm. I have mastered what that looks like on a patient from tens of thousands of x-rays to the patient themselves. I count in increments of seven and then subtract or add 1mm or 3mm, whatever is necessary to maintain accuracy with each and every visit. I also let the patient know so they can learn and understand their own body and its imbalances.

Body work is a very personalized event between two individuals. You must be extremely comfortable and exert tremendous trust in order to break through some blocks that you've guarded and protected for decades so you can reach new, higher goals for your health than you've ever experienced before. There are many obstacles, from your own fear, an unkept or mismanaged clinic, difficulty parking and excessive wait times to not-so-nice staff and personality conflicts with the doctor, etc. that can get in the way. Make sure these are all assessed before making your selection.

Once you have found someone you are comfortable working with, opt in for the full exam and x-rays. The doctor should be efficient in marking and measuring x-rays accurately. The three most important measurements are the difference of height between the right and the left top of the pelvis, your sacral base angle, and how much forward head posture you have in your neck. These are usually the largest imbalances in the body that need to be corrected the most. Thus, they are the focus of my S.E.T. program. If there are lateral curvatures seen on x-ray, your doctor should show you how to lie on a fulcrum on your side at the apex of the curve to accelerate correction. For the sake of simplicity, we will keep them out of the mix in this book and reserve them for clinical expertise.

Naturally there are many details we have missed in this book and in my S.E.T. Program design. For example, which exercises are best for structural change utilizing the torso and lower back muscles, etc. Suffice it to say, I am confident with what I have revealed and know that utilizing the program mapped out in this book will, without a doubt, correct a majority of your imbalances and change the structure of your physical frame to a better ergonomically correct position. It is imperative that you work closely with your health care professional while implementing this program and do not rely solely upon the merits outlined herein alone.

If everyone in the world followed the outlines with in the pages of this book, I promise you there would be less pain, muscle spasms, structural problems, and overall health issues in the given population, which would result in fewer personal injuries, workers' compensation claims, and visits to the emergency room, increasing the overall better health of the individual and the community.

So in the words of one of my favorite actors, Kelsey Grammer from the TV show *Frazier*, "Well then, off you go," my friends. Live Well & Rock On!

CONCLUSION

Hope that you have enjoyed reading my book.

This was truly an inspired labor of love and it is an honor to help in your journey ahead.

I know many of you still have a lot of unanswered questions. This book is finite in its material.

I vow to create YouTube videos to show exactly how to do these maneuvers with other variables.

My only hope is that this book in some little way has empowered you to a healthier you.

We all suffer aches and pains at some point throughout our lives. It's part of our human experience.

May this book teach you proper protocols to kick start you on your path of healing.

These are just a few tips that I have learned on my own journey and they have helped me tremendously!

I have spent many days on the floor stuck and screaming in pain without any aid from a professional.

I was forced to learn how to work with my own body utilizing my knowledge of how I work on others.

MORE BOOKS BY STATEN

This book is actually the second book I have written. I was encouraged by one of my publishers to release this book first. The first book I wrote is titled "Transitions: Coping in a Cracked-Up World." It is my remarkable life history, memoirs and experiences that are truly awe inspiring and almost unbelievable that so many things could happen to one person in a single lifetime. At fifty-six years old I have lived in fifty four houses in eight different states. I have been married six times.

I have been in almost every type of natural disaster and survived, from hurricanes, tornados, earthquakes and floods. I've experienced 9 near death events and been in situations where others died around me but I survived. I was homeless at seventeen years old and finished high school on my own. Incredibly I have persevered through addiction and beat that Goliath and have five years sober. I will do my best to get this other book on the shelves sometime in late 2020.

ABOUT THE AUTHOR

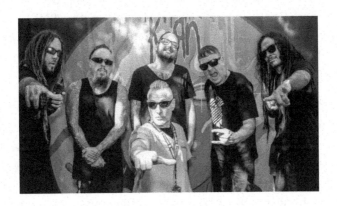

Dr. Staten Medsker, Jr is the wearer of many hats. He is the president of Mobile Chiropractic & Massage and Rockndoc Recording Studio in Seattle, Washington. He the founder of 2 bands, IRON ROD and Rockndoc and the Back Bones.

In Idaho he graduated from Lewiston High School in 1981. As an ordained Priest and Elder he served a mission for the Church of Jesus Christ of Latter Day Saints from 1982-1984 in Texas and Louisiana. His studies in pre-med were in Houston, Seattle and California. 1989-1992 he was class president at Life Chiropractic College West and as a musician performed in numerous shows and events. 1993 he was a guest panelist on the afternoon TV show "Town Meeting." During this time he wrote, directed and stared in 4 TV commercials.

His first publication was in Fortune Magazine on March 22, 1993. He continued his post education for 2 years in the CCSP (Certified Chiropractic Sports Physician) seminars. As a guest lecturer he taught at the Whole Life Expo and at Renton Vo-Tech College. He studied and received his certification as a Yoga instructor at the Yoga Barn in Bellevue, WA. He also studied personal training in the CSCS program (Certified Sports and Conditioning Specialist) and in the RNT program (Rebok Neuromuscular Training). In 1995 he began his car racing hobby and became the International Race Drivers Club novice driver of the year.

He became a member in 1996 of International Who's Who of Entrepreneurs and the Holistic Health Network. In 1997 he released his first CD as the band IRON ROD. He was also awarded a proclamation from the mayor of the City of Bellevue, Washington for his role in the education of our youth in health, safety and community awareness with "Kids Day America." He has appeared in numerous Journals and Newspapers, even making the front page four times.

He transitioned to Salt Lake City, UT in 2000 and 2001 to 2003 was a judge for the Miss Teen Utah pageants. While there, Dr. Medsker reformed his band IRON ROD and won the slot to play at the 2002 Winter Olympics. He was the chiropractor for the pro soccer team Salt Lake City Real (Blitz) and wrote his first musical titled "Hind Sight," (Non Published.) In 2002 he passed the audition and ended up as the host of "Club TV for six months."

Following his passion for TV and music, Dr. Medsker moved to Nashville, TN in 2006. In 2007 he hosted the reality TV show "The Experts" which never aired. He continued with a successful practice and in 2012 became a lecturer for the Tennessee Department of Health where he was also the lead medical volunteer for the Country Music Marathon.

His father, Staten Medsker, Jr. suffered a stroke in 2014 and Dr. Medsker returned to Seattle to care for his father. Upon returning to Seattle he re-released his first CD with IRON ROD which shot straight to number 1 on the Reverbnation charts and remained there for the next 5 years. Dr Medsker became a board member and singer for the Seattle Ensign Symphony and Chorus from 2015-2017.

In 2016 Dr. Medsker created the entity Adjustment-Manipulation Census. An international program to obtain the most accurate count of manipulations in the world. This was in conjunction registering with the Guinness World Records where he also attempted to adjust the most people in a single day. 2016-2018 he was the Emcee for the LLS Columbia Tower Firefighters Stair Climb.

In the last thirty years Dr. Medsker has been the chiropractor to over 300 famous musicians from bands like Bad Company, Def Leppard, The Eagles, Scorpions, Journey, Pink, Foreigner, Queensryche, Heart, Tool, Ted Nugent, Telsa, Weird Al, The Grateful Dead, Iron Maiden, and Ronny James Dio to name a few.

Dr. Medsker currently resides in Bellevue, Washington with his amazing wife Courtney and their 3-year-old daughter Presley. Dr. Medsker changed the name of his band to Rockndoc and the Back Bones and is in the middle of recording his second album which consist of a collaboration of over 50 famous musicians that have been his patients over the last thirty years.

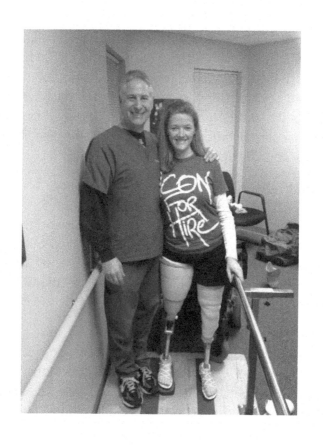

ACKNOWLEDGMENTS

Thank you, God, for always being there for me. Rescuing me when I needed it. Blessing me and inspiring me to create such beautiful music and keeping me in tune while I heal others. Especially for giving me my gifts of healing through touch, music and the spoken word.

Huge thank you to my wife Courtney for supporting and believing in me and teaching me how to be patient, responsible and grounded. You are my beacon of purity and charity.

Thank YOU, the reader, for investing your time and money to support me in this book.

Thank you to my amazing mother, Bonnie Butz who taught me how to laugh and see the light side of troubles and teaching me how to serve others (especially the homeless) by example.

Thank you to Jo Fasen for writing the amazing forward to this book.

Thank you to my dad, Staten Sr. who has shown me how to master endurance and giving me the gene's for creating. Your legacy lives on through me!

Thank you to all the amazing friends that I have worked with over the past forty plus years. Each of them has made a great impact on my life.

So grateful for all of my patients over the years that have taught me so much how to love, heal and serve. I love each and every one of you for sharing my journey. All of you have taught me how to be the best student.

CONTACT INFORMATION

Staten (Rockndoc) can be reached at Rockndoc4@yahoo.com

Listen to Staten's music at
https://www.reverbnation.com/ironrodtheband

Follow Staten on Facebook at:

> Personal Page:
> https://www.facebook.com/drstaten.medskerjr

> Official Fan Page:
> https://www.facebook.com/CEOdrStatenMedsker/

> Business Page: https://www.facebook.com/Mobile-Kairo-Healings-854069437960912/

> Adman Censes:
> https://www.facebook.com/search/top/?q=2017%20Adjustment-Manipulation%20Census&epa=SEARCH_BOX

Connect with Staten on LinkedIn at:
https://www.linkedin.com/in/dr-staten-medsker-jr-6505ba25/

TESTIMONIALS

Best Chiropractor I have ever met. Staten taught me how to hold my back straight, roll my shoulders back and adjust my hips and get that natural curve back in my neck. In short, Staten taught me how to listen to my body and take better care of it!

A. Watson, Seattle, WA

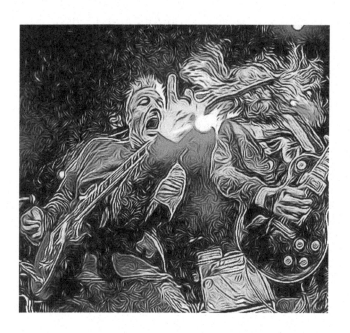

FEEDBACK REQUEST

Please leave a review for my book as I would greatly appreciate your feedback.

If for some reason you did not enjoy the book then please contact me at Rockndoc4@yahoo.com to discuss options prior to leaving a negative review and please feel free to let me know how the book can be improved.

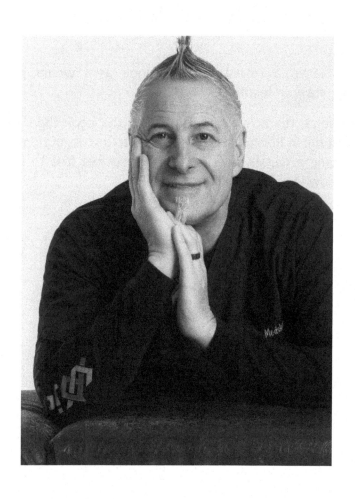

Made in USA - North Chelmsford, MA
1363238_9781734805345
06.04.2023 1330